## More Praise for *Keeping Room*

You might not suspect a book that begins with cancer, covid, hypoxia, nuclear medicine, and the ER to be hopeful. But after a long and hard narrative through health issues, nightmares, and gun violence, we find ourselves in the Pine Barrens after a hurricane, or ruminating over untended gardens. Wallace leaves us not with loss but with "a bending toward hope," and days of reclamation. There are mourning doves and wild clover, salamanders and a "spit of woodland" – as if the mere presence of the natural world may heal. "There is sweetness here in this year of pain and solitude," an attentive to the small things of the world. These are poems written out of hard struggle. But in the end, through her music and her art, Wallace leads us home, with heart, hope, and healing, to witness chefs making breakfast and bakers baking – to live, to eat.

— **Sean Thomas Dougherty**, author of *Death Prefers the Minor Keys*

# KEEPING ROOM

## ANN E. WALLACE

Nixes Mate Books
Allston, Massachusetts

Copyright © 2026 Ann E. Wallace

Book design by d'Entremont
Cover photograph used with permission.

All rights reserved. This book or any portion thereof may not be reproduced or used in any manner whatsoever without the express written permission of the publisher except for the use of brief quotations in a book review or scholarly journal.

ISBN 978-1-949279-63-4

Nixes Mate Books
PO Box 1179
Allston, MA 02134
nixesmate.pub

*Not knowing when the dawn will come,
I open every door.*

— Emily Dickinson

# CONTENTS

| | |
|---|---|
| Latent | 3 |
| The Keeping Room | 4 |
| After the Accident | 5 |
| On Graduating from College with an Ovarian Cancer Diagnosis | 6 |
| Tendrils | 7 |
| Kindred | 8 |
| Ready to Live | 10 |
| When the Forsythia Blooms | 11 |
| Master Class with Alice Waters | 12 |
| Lesson in Danger | 13 |
| Nightmare with Hypoxia | 14 |
| Emergency Room Visits in March 2020 | 15 |
| Cleared to Leave | 17 |
| Another Nightmare | 19 |
| This Morning in Nuclear Medicine | 20 |
| Another Nightmare | 22 |
| Afternoon at the Neurologist | 23 |
| This Fragile Cusp | 25 |
| The Baker | 27 |
| Another Nightmare | 30 |
| Breakfast, Compromised | 31 |
| Another Nightmare | 32 |
| Standing in Emily's Garden | 34 |
| Upon Reflection on the Spring Calendar | 35 |
| A Small Respite | 37 |
| Lesson in Trust | 39 |
| Love Note | 40 |
| The Day Another Gun Law Is Repealed | 41 |
| How to Handle a Leak | 42 |
| A Small Palm on the Glass | 44 |
| Lesson in Care | 46 |

| | |
|---|---|
| August Elegy | 47 |
| September Walk in the New Jersey Pine Barrens after Hurricane Helene | 48 |
| In Anticipation of an Elegy | 49 |
| Clear Cut | 50 |
| Jersey City Facebook Group, A Cento | 51 |
| The sky in my backyard is opening | 52 |
| Looming | 53 |
| Lesson in Flying | 54 |
| Such a Perfect Ecosystem | 55 |
| Referral | 57 |
| Supple | 58 |
| Overloaded | 60 |
| Accounting | 61 |
| Lesson in Survival | 62 |
| Reserves | 63 |
| A Final Offering | 64 |
| Anne Frank's Classmates | 67 |
| The Funeral Director, Spring 2020 | 68 |
| Hoboken, November 2020 | 70 |
| In State | 72 |
| The Alchemy of Crisis | 74 |
| Health Care Proxy | 75 |
| Tidal Forces | 78 |
| Tax Season | 80 |
| Spring Morning | 82 |
| Assisted Breathing | 83 |
| After the Book Fair, New Jersey City University | 84 |
| Paper Trails | 85 |
| How to End | 86 |
| Failure | 87 |
| How I Live Now | 88 |
| Bending Toward Hope | 89 |

# KEEPING ROOM

I

# LATENT

A body can feel only
one pain at a time.

The brain meters it out,
flips a switch,
receives an aching
signal from one direction,
not another.

One pain at a time,
the body is kept safe.

## THE KEEPING ROOM

There comes a time when the phones
are powered down, the shutters pulled tight.
Within the keeping room, we worry.
We wait.

When life is reduced to the smallest
motions, to the thrumming pain of leaving,
unheard, invisible to all but those of us
here gathered, we know but cannot bear
to concede, hope's time has passed.

# AFTER THE ACCIDENT

I found the mourning dove on Saturday
as I was working in my yard. I shuddered,
took a deep breath and half looked away

as I nudged it with the dustpan's edge
into the bag of debris and weeds
I hauled to the curb for pickup.

Hours later a car drove too fast. No, a driver
drove too fast, or distracted, or both.
She slammed into my car filled with people

I love, yet she did not kill us. We extracted
ourselves from the crumpled mess and left
it there in the road for someone to tow away.

Two days later, I stepped into my yard again,
filled the empty feeder for the anxious birds
I had watched hover as I lay silent, recovering.

I found a tiny baby bird, lifeless on the chair
beneath the cherry tree that held an empty nest
hidden high within its branches.

## ON GRADUATING FROM COLLEGE WITH AN OVARIAN CANCER DIAGNOSIS

The spring I turned twenty-two
I finished college and learned to track
my bloodwork the way others count their calories.

My doctor didn't need to write the order
for the nurses. I could rattle it off –
CBC    CA125    AFP

I would count the days until my refrigerator
was restocked with bags of chemo, my bathroom
sharps container stuffed with spent needles.

Blood type: *B positive*, like a reminder.
I knew that too. And tried to be.
My home nurses in their thick gloves

and blue hazmat gowns tended to all
that went in and out of my veins, made sure
the hurried lab techs did not overfill

their glass vials with my blood –
*They don't need that much.*
*But you do.*

# TENDRILS

I stoop to loosen a thread of wild clover woven tight
through my spotty lawn, and recall the morning
I knelt on my small patch of yard and pulled

stretch after stretch of unwanted stem, made room
for grass in the barren spaces, my belly eight months full,
pulling, pulling at home in the Jersey August heat.

I vowed to yank out every last bit. I rarely tug
at the thin tendrils these days – I no longer need
a soft surface for kiddie pools and yard toys.

My lawn's future is short now, as I welcome
the spread and creep of native flowers, but the green
threads winding across the earth remain a portal

into the summer before motherhood, before I learned
that disruption and love equal joy.

## KINDRED

Sometimes I think I must have spent a lifetime
as a girl searching alone and in silence for toads

and salamanders, hoisting stones and peering
between blades of grass in the woods across the street,

where my four brothers, all older, dug for antique
bottles and other treasures, where later they stashed

their illicit magazines in the adjacent cemetery. I could just
tell you that I adored the smallest animals hiding out

of sight and under my nose in the woods across the street.
But then you would have no idea the intensity of a small girl

who spirited each hot and humid day away from her family
of boys, who found delight in the hunt for creatures

smaller than she, creatures with the innate good sense to stay
tucked away as rough siblings staked their claim

on that spit of woodland, a girl who loved bumpy toads
the color of dry New England earth and the slick backs

of salamanders with their finely wrought toes so dearly
that she would hold them in her palms for just a moment

then gently place them back in their homes, satisfied
that they had survived another day.

## READY TO LIVE

The campus was always the most
vibrant in springtime –

forsythia spraying unwieldy
shoots of yellow against the verdant

landscape of greens popping bright
after weeks of mud and groaning

as students sleep-walked through finals.
I saw it all again through my 22-year-old eyes –

my final campus season of exams,
surgery, and chemo,

a somber beginning set against
nature's near-neon boast.

# WHEN THE FORSYTHIA BLOOMS

My father once told me the time
to put down grass seed

is when the forsythia blooms.
I noticed those scraggly yellow buds

on the roadside the other day,
the same week my backyard cherry tree

began sprouting soft sprays of pink.
And so it is time to tend

to the winter-trodden earth
of my garden, to kneel in the damp soil

to till it by hand, thin out old growth
and pull stones that surfaced in cold

upheavals, in preparation for spring.
But I am still heaving rocks myself

and carrying the cold weight of winter
that has held on tight and long, as I gasp

for air and kick toward the surface where
delicate flowers have begun to blossom.

# MASTER CLASS WITH ALICE WATERS

In the kitchen, she speaks in a halting voice,
as if she knows words interrupt the conversation
between hands, nose, mouth and radicchio,

radish, turnip. She holds fingerlings, greens,
almonds, tilts her head *I'm thinking I will make...*
the idea arrives, lips part into a smile, eyes brighten,

*yes, that will be perfect.* I want to be there with her
between stove and wood-topped island, pounding
garlic into pungent pulp, awakening olives

in the iron skillet, splashing oil onto fresh chicory.
Her fingers work mounds of produce
into flavors that spark quiet sighs of delight.

## LESSON IN DANGER

Why would a hawk pause to take short station
in my city spit of a yard? The fence-top perch

grants dominion over the entire gridded block of green,
and under the sharp eye of predator, a small world

of sparrows, cardinals, and squirrels flee for safety –
where, across the street? Over the town line?

For days, the humming yard, the brimming bird
feeder, sit quiet. With a flash of massive wing

and an arrogant glare, the hawk claimed this territory
then moved to fresher ground, yet its dark shadow

lingers over the precious plot of life outside my window.
Today, a few anxious sparrows return, flit in and out

of the dogwood, peck at kernels and seeds,
and flap to safety as I approach the pane to watch.

## NIGHTMARE WITH HYPOXIA

At night in the car, my daughter
and I have a meal delivery for Konstantin,
alone tending the unending barrage
of covid deceased in a desolate warehouse.

Our brakes give out on a clover
leaf exit, we miss the turn, careen
out of control, fly past our destination,
pick up speed on the empty streets.

Rocketing through red lights
flashing bright in the dark deserted city
faster,    faster,
on course to hit a building, a lamp post,
an abandoned car, something.

It will happen. It is only a matter
of time.

## EMERGENCY ROOM VISITS IN MARCH 2020

When they turned the pediatric emergency room
into a COVID triage area in the early days,

decals of monkeys with curling tails,
loping elephants, spotted giraffes grazed

the walls. The doctor who took my vitals
was tired, hadn't seen his kids in two weeks.

The hospital prepared to admit me, then sent
me home after two rounds of bloodwork and testing.

They needed the bed. Three days later, I returned
on my 50$^{th}$ birthday, barely conscious,

bypassed the children's unit, and was wheeled inside
where the serious cases were handled.

The aide hesitated to help me onto the bed,
offered a gloved hand only after I pleaded,

and my new doctor would not step inside
my curtain. He poked his masked face

through the gap in the fabric to ask
my cell number. He wrote it on a Post-it

and backed away like from a caged tiger.
I never received his call.

## CLEARED TO LEAVE

My face is pale and splotchy when my ex-
husband picks me up at home, like death
blooms within me. The weather, April

dreary. Jason drives me to the emergency room –
my third hospital this spring. I wear a pink
woolen cap, loop my oxygen line around my ears,

tuck it behind my glasses, hook the cannula
under my nose. I lug the tank inside
and sit in a folding chair in the makeshift

waiting room – the department had been under
renovation when the virus hit. The work
on the building has stopped. The work of saving

lives has not. My doctor called ahead
for a lung scan. The ER doctor takes my blood
and vitals but never orders the scan.

I rest in my thin, faded hospital gown,
in the overwhelmed ER, so much like the others,
each one unique in its chaos. Cleared to leave,

I dress slowly, layer by layer – shirt and pants,
sweater, jacket, hat. Untethered from the hospital
oxygen, reconnected to my emergency supply

from home, I hoist the tank. Alone, undirected,
I stumble through the halls, carry my heavy load,
search for the unmarked exit. Outside in the cold,

I realize I left my glasses on my hospital bed.
They are gone. Per pandemic policy, thrown
into the trash with all other personal effects.

# ANOTHER NIGHTMARE

A starless night, a storm broils,
jerks me out of bed. My old house
shudders and lists.

Sharp winds whistle through the walls,
wrench the double front doors
from their ancient hinges.

I steel myself in the empty doorway,
grip the wood framing, arms spread taut
against nature's force like a captain at sea.

High above the leaf-tattered street,
I watch the doors of my house loft and bob
on the gusting gales, into the wet night.

The front steps, the porch ripped away,
my battered house teeters and steadies.
It holds strong.

My body pulling, pushing
like a sail against nature's wrath,
I stand watch in the raging darkness.

My daughters sleep within.

# THIS MORNING IN NUCLEAR MEDICINE

I consider the orange pill tucked inside the blue pouch
buried deep within my purse. I am too tired to fish it out
and wash it down with a swig of warm water, even if it holds
the power to stop my weary head from pounding.

Nearby, my daughter sleeps inside the NM 830 machine
that tracks radioactive movement inside her stomach, a bland
microwaved egg churning, breaking down, its steady journey
recorded and projected on the computer screen across the room.

*All I ask is that if I die, don't save me.*
A woman's voice from behind the curtained machine next to ours
pleads and a man responds with gentle instructions, and, I can tell
though I cannot see, with gentle touch.

*We need to get you on the table. I have your oxygen.*
I hear him position the woman for a sequence of lung scans,
a test I was scheduled to have four years ago, so sick like my neighbor,
but, for some hazy failure in communication, never did.

The man guides her arms above her head for the next image,
then down again. Her voice is small –

*I hurt so much.*

*I do too, Patricia. I do too,*
I want to say. I want to dull the sharp volume of instructive voices,
the plaintive cries of the woman, the terror-filled shrieks of a toddler
pulsing from behind a curtain somewhere down the hall.

I want to pull my daughter from the yawning mouth of the NM 830,
pull her from another morning in the bowels of a hospital,
the same hospital where, the virus raging, I was once covered head to toe
in a sheet like a corpse, *like a corpse, Patricia,* and wheeled inside for scans.

Wary of the turbulence the pill in my purse might call forth
as I wait two hours for the scrambled egg to digest
inside my sleeping daughter's stomach, I close my eyes and sink
into the pulsing, pulsing pain of this place.

*We just want to make you comfortable.*
The frail woman cannot hear the man though his voice
is loud and also kind. Her hearing is weak,
her hips ache, her lungs burn.

Finally, she is done. She is alive.
*I could never have done this without you. Jimmy, you're a keeper.*
The woman is wheeled away, away from this place
before my daughter wakes.

A new patient I cannot see is rolled into the empty place
behind the curtain behind my back,
and the pain gripping the base of my skull softens
in the silence.

# ANOTHER NIGHTMARE

I can feel it still –
the muddy suck beneath my feet,
soggy pine planks sinking,
sinking, where they lie,
into the dirt.

My kitchen is slowly pulled
toward the center of the earth,
stove teetering, water lines
leaking, walls askew.

At the edge of the room,
my toes curl and grip,
find purchase, resist the force,
hold tight. I slowly back away.

# AFTERNOON AT THE NEUROLOGIST

The tech lays out the bundle
of wires before joining them
one by one, with a dab of paste,
to my daughter's scalp,
until her head is covered
with goop and nodes
and plastic-coated strands.

As kids, we used to covet and hoard
such bright-colored wires. I can't
even remember why. The red,
white, and black threads I swiped
from my father's workshop
weren't worth much in the scheme
of schoolyard values next to the rainbow
hues other girls bought new
at the hardware store. What accessories
we made with these strands
is now lost to me, but the colors.

They lured us the way narrow pastel
and jewel-toned satin ribbons did
a year or two later, when we wove them
around and through the bands

of our barrettes, leaving long
smooth tails to hang loose in our hair.

We wove them like the technician
wraps the band of white gauze
around, around my daughter's head
and leaves the trail of wires –
red, orange, blue, yellow, and more –
like a braid down her back, bundled
and covered in a cotton sheath,
ready for three days of testing.
I can no longer see the colors.

# THIS FRAGILE CUSP

There is sweetness here
    in this year of pain and solitude,

a foggy burrowing, punctuated
    by sparks of clarity, of laughter.

Sixteen here is a year of interruption,
    of breath, words,

movement suspended beyond reach,
    a break in the steady march

away from childhood,
    a post-viral hibernation

at home, of sickbed days and silence,
    but the gift of mother-

daughter time is found here too,
    on this fragile cusp

of adulthood as each day cycles
    through appointments,

sleep, pain, so much pain, and not
   much else, ever circling

toward, away,
   and toward, recovery.

# THE BAKER

With a sweep of her arm, she applies the blade
to the crumb-coated cake, polishes the surface

shiny clean like plaster and charts a course
on the buttercream, leaning in close to map

the threads of liquid chocolate. She weighs
a loaded tube, gives a slight squeeze to fill

the nozzle, bends with the squinting eye
of a scientist to her microscope, and sets

the plate spinning, the needle touching down
as chocolate pools and glistens still like glass.

I watch, holding my breath as my daughter
touches the plastic tip to the smooth wet

surface, releases dark-pearled drips, controls
each stream that cascades down the iced tiers,

strand after strand beading to a precise stop.
The young baker turns her table, steady,

drip upon drip, until a bubble of air
bursts the tube, gushing warm ganache

down the pristine cake to puddle at its base.
She jumps back and drops her failed tools.

It is ruined. With a mother's deep urge
to assure that all is not lost, I survey

the wide flow of chocolate, the dented
cake, the stain of spilt icing. Yes, it may be.

As I assess, she sets her shoulders square,
crouches eye level with the damage, gives

the slightest nod and returns to work.
With palette knife and towel, warm water

and icing, she scrapes and smooths, adds new drips
and achieves the illusion of perfection.

It is saved. But I see the subtle slump
in her shoulders as she secures her work

onto the tray, closes the lid, and holds
the cake steady as I navigate potholed

winter roads for a safe delivery.
Upon the party table, the bright glaze

of ganache catches light, refracted onto
the baker. The flaw, though hidden,

is not forgotten, and she deflects the glow
of praise for a less than perfect cake.

## ANOTHER NIGHTMARE

I must navigate the rutted dirt road
through the verdant wild forest,
carry my daughters to safety,
to help, away from our viral home.

Miles in, so far from the familiar,
the way is flooded from weeks
of spring's heavy rain. The car's tires
suck and stick in clay-like mud.

The wooded passage too narrow
for turning back, we inch
our way forward, lost and alone
in the deepening dark.

# BREAKFAST, COMPROMISED

Chef Alice Waters does not share
her breakfast secrets, but as I whisk

cream of wheat into simmering milk,
I think of her kitchen, warm with copper

and wood, where slow and simple reign.
I think a spoon of homemade cherry

preserves, a wedge of sweet Jersey peach
could finish my homely porridge. I can see her

cutting a slice with paring knife, sniffing
for freshness, the spread of smile as she holds

the bit of fruit before her, as if to say, *oh yes,
perfect.* I savor the moment of wonder as I eat

my breakfast standing alone at my island,
scrolling, hungry, on my phone.

## ANOTHER NIGHTMARE

The viral barrage goes on,
night after night –
storm waters rise
high and higher,
the city sinks away,
my solitary house
grows tall, sprouts
new floors
above the floods.

I climb up, up,
up to safety,
hurry against the water
always seeping in,
to wait out these acts of God
above the waterline
alone,   alone,
                alone.

II

## STANDING IN EMILY'S GARDEN

The kousa dogwood, alone
and small, arches its branches,

under the towering oaks. Its
dimpled red berries, delicate,

dangle from short stems – all
it takes is slight pressure

from an intruder to burst its soft
shell. And yet, the tree stands

tall in its own skin, and its seeds
sink into the welcome earth.

## UPON REFLECTION ON THE SPRING CALENDAR

As showy as it is,
April is a trash month.

I mean, not just because
it is all gaudiness and mud,

no, the real offense
is that it is so damn bright,

year after year – I mean,
just look at the ungainly

forsythia spattered with a yellow
so loud few people can wear,

let alone a scraggly roadside bush –
and so wretched. Maybe

it's personal, my fury,
but tell me it's not justified –

when April brings an onslaught
of storms and pain and hospitals

each year to me
and mine.

Truly, I prefer
a more humble month.

## A SMALL RESPITE

What I want today is the voice of Alice Waters
inviting me into her warm kitchen, to select greens,

imbibe their sweet fragrance, shred them bit by bit
into an earthen bowl, toss in oil, vinegar, a pinch

of good salt, with able hands, to partake in the ancient
art of crafting a meal with care and patience.

Today, I do not want the flash and chime of text
after text after text, of email flooding my inbox,

all day, all night, the grip pulling, tight and tighter,
in my chest when I can't keep up.

What I want today is small –
energy to tend my garden, to pull, trim, snip

the loud and wilted old growth, last year's detritus
that taunts me now as I wake and gaze

through the picture window, to scoop a small grave
for the baby bird that fell from her nest in the cherry tree

and pat cool soil over her fragile wings, to fill planters
and beds and sit back, exhausted, and watch

through the glass as sparrows, finches, and their songbird
brethren flit and vie for short respite at my backyard feeder.

# LESSON IN TRUST

I have fallen
for the gray cat
who has made a place
for herself in my yard.

I have offered my garden,
tucked away places to shelter and hide,
and my door left ajar for the girl
with the faint stripes and the damp
eyes who waits for me in the morning.

Smaller and more timid
than the jowly tom who used to nap
in the sunny corner of the patio
and ran when I came too close,
this soul will allow me to offer
regular meals and medicine,
fresh water and soft words,
even a name – Clementine,
slow blinking at me as she lounges
on my garden chair.

She trusts me, but not enough
to let me give her a home.

## LOVE NOTE

I did not see the granola bar until I was at work,
rummaging through my bag for lipstick

or a tissue. My daughter must have slipped it
into my purse as I hurried to make lunches,

brush snarled hair, secure small feet into shoes,
zip stubborn jackets, grab my brimming bags

and theirs, in the harried moments before
herding us all out the door.

The small pink Post-it poked from inside
my leather bag, pasted onto the foil wrapper,

reminding me in the wobbly letters
of second grade to eat my lunch.

# THE DAY ANOTHER GUN LAW IS REPEALED

I see my first tulip of the season,
the bud still green, closed up tight,

showing just a blush of ripening red,
and the bleeding hearts begin

unfurling their fragile pink flowers
in the community garden at the end

of my street. The warm damp air,
the drops of color, the too-sweet

scent of hyacinth smother me.
Blooms spring from the concrete

and in narrow patches of light
and green between buildings.

Tended or not, brazen flowers show up
each spring and claim their light.

# HOW TO HANDLE A LEAK

My daughters and I live in a leaky
old house. The three of us have

learned how to handle a plumbing
emergency, to spring into action,

sop up the mess, cut the water lines,
track the source, mend the seams.

This is what women do.
We live in bodies that bleed,

are vulnerable, that give life
but also betray, and we have

passed down the fortitude
to handle leaks and other messes.

There is wisdom in our living,
and we know how to act

when a leak is sprung, exposing
the ill intentions of those

who do not live in our bodies,
those who spout outrage

at the egregious betrayal –
as if they know what betrayal is –

of being caught with the pipe
cutters in their bloody hands.

While they sputter and point fingers,
we – the women – are gathering

our tools, our rage and our ballots,
like we have so many times before.

And we are ready to fight
for our freedom.

## A SMALL PALM ON THE GLASS

A girl in Newtown crouched
so long and so hard, in the corner
of her hushed classroom –

the way children do when terror
floods their bodies – that she cracked
two vertebrae.

We call her a survivor.

The fissures healed
but her back still aches.
It ached as she crouched, still,

ten years later in Michigan,
as her college classmates were shot,
killed.

Her body remembers.

A small girl on a bus in Nashville
placed her open palm
against the window pane,

her open mouth wrenched,
her open eyes streaming,
her silent wail caught on camera –

we've seen these images before
and we know how to look away –
as she was delivered to safety.

To her parents
waiting,    waiting,
waiting.

We count her
among the survivors.
My youngest was six

when Newtown's six-year-olds died.
She was safe in a different school,
in a different state.

But my body, held tight for so long,
remembers.

## LESSON IN CARE

When Connie was four, or maybe five, she suggested
we create a sanctuary in the attic, so raccoons

on the street would know to come in and be safe,
but of course the raccoons on the street,

and in the garden, and on the cliff side, already
knew to shimmy up the side of the house,

to the porch roof, and past the second floor,
to squeeze through an invisible fissure

under the eaves, where they would find safety.
I think she knew this too

and was simply asking me to leave them
alone.

# AUGUST ELEGY

Some people grow tired of summer
by August – they long for the cooling
night, the sun's slip low in the sky,
see scorched grass and look skyward
for turning leaves.

Not me. I soak up the hot, hot sun,
invite it to warm me to my core.
I want to hold August close
as my grown children tick another year
off the calendar, ever cycling

further from the song and skip
of parties and piñatas, kiddie pools
and fireflies cupped in our palms,
and have another go at getting it right.

## SEPTEMBER WALK IN THE NEW JERSEY PINE BARRENS AFTER HURRICANE HELENE

I might tell you about my long walk
in the forest, about the scent of pine,
of cedar, of sandy loam on the soft

wooded floor. I could bring you
there, into silence, into the wind's
creak and whirl on the empty trail,

into the shallow stream's slow
meander. I would want you to see
the colors, the wild blueberry bushes

turning rich sienna, the ruddy bark
of evergreens, the light soil
beneath brittle brown needles,

the bright azure sky. What I would
give to share the golden luck of this
September day, so mild despite the wet

and stormy forecast. But how could I
offer such beauty, when my mind
and yours, is south, where the weather

we did not get stalled, made land fall,
bridges and roads collapsed, and houses
slipped with ease into roiling rivers?

# IN ANTICIPATION OF AN ELEGY

I began mourning
my garden last year
when news broke

of the large building to rise
behind my house. Neighbors,
we fought for light, for life, for trees.

We won a stay of execution –
I mean, a rejection
by the planning board.

But it is only a matter
of time. Our leaders, they choose
to not understand

that trees and plants mean
so much here, in this city,
sustain birds and other creatures,

like us, who scratch the soil
and take shelter beneath
the vanishing canopy.

# CLEAR CUT

In these chill and dormant months, pleasure
is tucked away, and wonder brews and thrums
invisible, beneath winter's cloak. I do not walk
as much as I would like, or as I did in the fall,

when the weather was fair, the rewards of summer
still ablaze. In the bare space of the new year, I pull
on my woolen coat, step outside and down the street.
Clouds sit heavy over Manhattan across the river,

the air held still. And in the park, where asters bloom
in late summer and bees suck the September nectar
doing their quiet buzzing work with ease and without
distraction, pulling pollen so the rain garden will seed

and flower next year, I see a swath of native garden
cut clear and naked by city workers who could not see
emergent spring pulsing within crisp seed pods
or under browned and fallen leaves.

Gone. All gone.

Scythed and uprooted, the frail bedraggled refuse
tossed into piles, and hauled off as so much trash,
leaving us to ask when we might ever have the wisdom
to step away and let wonder bloom in spite of us.

# JERSEY CITY FACEBOOK GROUP, A CENTO

Most of you don't know how trees grow and it shows.

Google is your friend.
Asphalt is porous.

Art – a baby tree locked in tar.

Talk about weed prevention.

Is that City mulch?

Sure, they ran out of cement.

It probably looks better than it was before.
It keeps the dogs from fertilizing the trees.

Efficiency. If it works it works.

Art – because Jersey City hates trees.
Now trending JC. Why?

Next it will be a fake tree.

How many trees have been planted
only to be left to die?

Btw, that's the size of a parking spot.
Just sayin'.

## THE SKY IN MY BACKYARD IS OPENING

Up. I've been watching as the plum tree extends
its arms and breathes *finally*.

Large machines with claws, rollers in place
of wheels, rake at the ramshackle walls

of the neighboring garage, an eyesore to be sure
in this city where sharp prospectors are swift

to set such weary structures in their scopes
and level them, dust to dust.

If I listen closely, I can hear the birds swoop in,
fill the branches, their voices tender

against the crackle and roar of demolition.
I begin to mourn this brief opening

before the sky closes once again, when the ground
is laid bare and the developer's plans have yet

to rise from the page – bigger, taller –
in the back corner of my exposed garden.

The tree that now breathes in relief
has no idea the darkness coming.

# LOOMING

The noise is less deafening now —
the foundation has been laid and high walls

erected on my block. The construction
workers have moved inside, where they install

the systems, partitions, and finishes, out
of sight, that will make the monstrosity run.

The noise has quieted, but the damage
is set in concrete and will not be undone.

## LESSON IN FLYING

A pound and a half of feathers, beak,
and hollow bones swoop swift

on three-foot wings from the power line
to a dried out branch that cracks

and drops beneath the sudden load.
The Harris hawk, too young to know

his own slight bulk, or which trees
are alive and strong, alights only to fall,

again and again, with startled midair
saves, fast flapping to more solid

limbs. Spectators crane their necks,
spines straining and mouths agape.

They marvel at a bird of prey, still
learning the force of its weight.

## SUCH A PERFECT ECOSYSTEM

Yesterday I celebrated small things
in a room packed with people who oohed

when the entomologist told of the magnificence
of the spring beauty, a plant with pale pink blossoms

so petite and fleeting that most Jersey lawn
tenders miss them flickered through the grass.

I don't mean we long for or regret no longer seeing
them. I mean we don't see the flowers at all.

But they are not invisible, not to the mining bees
who light upon the tiny petals and coat

their fuzzy bellies with the sweet pink nectar
these beauties create just for them.

III

# REFERRAL

I would like to send you
to my cigarette-smoking

oncologist with her thick
accent and her sturdy

heels. She would get straight
to work, ignore distractions,

save your life. She would risk
it all for you, like she did for me –

with steely confidence, a plan
and a backup, for a patient too young

to be impressed. I wish you
could see my good doctor

and how she gave me these
decades before she was gone.

# SUPPLE

I listen to the pull of a cello's bow,
and whole notes rife with pain
lodge deep in my chest.

I know that beauty grows there,
where low tones resonate
within the swell of spruce.

I watch the rocking arm cradle
and release the sound, so smooth,
and I wonder when I developed

a stiff upper lip – that is not
a metaphor – meant to shelter
and brace against loss, the open book

of my face ossified from once
arching bow into steeled facade?
Long ago, when a body failed, piece

by piece, doctors called upon engineers
to design replacements, prosthetic hips
and knees fabricated from metal, on faith

that steel might stand in for pulsing marrow,
for living bone, as if engineers did not already
know that even bridges must be allowed to swell

and flex like music. Some experts believed
that tensile strength is what a body needs
and forgot that when we groan and stretch

dynamic, like strings over the warmth
of a cello's belly, pain and ache are given
voice within the beauty, and the sublime

will waft through the fine hairs,
bend and bow with the grace
of a supple wrist.

## OVERLOADED

Scientists discover
that death often comes by the chemo
not the cancer.

Well, of course.
Or, either. Or both.

Does it matter?

# ACCOUNTING

At the edge of fifty I was afraid
to look at the balance of my bank account,

to do the math of what was needed
to get from there to here, subtracting

from all I had squirreled away. I expected
to have more, a compiling, for it to have

added up to something I could cash in on,
but at fifty, the value of this life was not

in the books. No, I found it in my staccato,
hard-fought breath that pulsed and paused,

that stuttered but, determined, kept
pushing me on and on, to this far shore.

## LESSON IN SURVIVAL

This year's cherry blossoms
grow directly from their trunks,
bypass the leggy limbs to pull
straight from the marrow.
Trees know to adapt in times
of crisis. Like us, as we hold
close what is young and fragile.

# RESERVES

You cooked the ravioli, warmed
the marinara on my stove, plated it all

just so, added a sprinkle of cheese
and placed the bowl before me with a smile.

I did not know for many months that you
do not like ravioli or even that particular sauce,

but you had offered to cook, to conjure
a meal from the pitiful stores of my pantry.

You had not bargained for the truth of my self-
proclaimed empty reserves, yet undeterred, you pulled

jars from shelves, searched the fridge and poured
yourself into making a meal out of nothing for me.

## A FINAL OFFERING

He brought the Entenmann's cookies
and Russian candies his grandmother loved,
to nestle in the crook of her arm
as she lay on his embalming table.

He spoke soft words and stopped to stroke her hair
every few hours over two or three long September days
before lifting her in his arms and placing her
to rest in the plain wooden casket.

He drove her to the cemetery, directed
the small group of mourners, and shoveled
mound after mound of earth in his shirtsleeves,
until the grave was filled.

When he was a boy in Brooklyn, she fed him
treats and with an abundance she
and two sisters had not known holed up
in a small apartment in wartime Riga.

At eighteen, excited to build a new life,
with city jobs and modern freedoms,
she left their countryside village,
their parents, three youngest sisters behind.

When Hitler stormed into Latvia, she learned
strength, would not crack in front
of sweet Rose, just fifteen,
or Basia, the oldest.

Only in the thick quiet of night, could she, Masha, twist
and turn, the knot of fear tightening. She'd heard
the rumors – neighbors were killing Jews in the villages.
Villages like her family's.

Only there, in bed, in the dark, could she sob
when the news reached the city – the Soviet Army
blew up a railway bridge as her family, on their way out,
to safety, traveled over. There were no survivors.

It was only there, in the dark, her body shook
and shuddered, her trust in the world
blasted along with the pilings and suspended
railbed into a million shards of shattered hope.

Decades later, to her lone grandson, born
to her only daughter, whom she had named
for bounty awaiting a fall, after the garden of Eden,
she offered the richest food –

pomegranates, from which she plucked each bloody seed,
and shrimp, deveined and presented in a fine glass dish,
pints of ice cream, the sweetest cookies –
without limit, served to him but not his friends.

Her grandson must not ever feel the losses
she had known in his gut. She needed to offer him
a fighting chance in a world where nothing
was guaranteed, and nothing promised.

Embarrassment and pleasure battled within
the grandson, but he learned that we must feed,
in abundance and without restraint, the ones we love,
store up the reserves for when they may be needed.

He offers his final gift to her, one not meant to be repaid,
placing the box of chocolates in her casket.

# ANNE FRANK'S CLASSMATES

The black and white photo of five-year-olds
looks like any Montessori class anywhere,
some children distracted, most smiling, one

girl in the foreground blurry with movement.
A teacher crouches low behind the desks
at the edge of the room, level with her students.

The gift in this image is that the children did not
know that room imbued with love was a capsule
that would not keep. Half the faces etched

by light and dark into that still image did not
survive the decade, extinguished into silence
at Auschwitz, at Sobibor, at Bergen-Belsen.

Most left no trace, no surviving parent to remember
their faces, their stumbles, their fears, no one
left to mourn the people they should have become.

## THE FUNERAL DIRECTOR, SPRING 2020

He bites his lower lip, clasps
his hands behind his back, and steels
his legs into a wide stance, knowing

one brimming tear holds power to unleash
the others welled up and waiting.
It used to be the unexpected

that disrupted his balance – the new suit
purchased two sizes too small
for a teen struck down in the road,

the calm words of a mother
to her grown child laid out before her, speaking
of tomorrow as if nothing had changed,

or the collapse and despair of another
who knew everything had.
But in these endless days of horror

when the pandemic envelops
and makes a home in our city –
when the morgues are overflowing,

and the bodies are stacked and held
three weeks for burial, when the caskets
are closed and families can not kiss

or send off their dear beloved – he works
in solitude, carrying the grief of legions.
He removes the tubes and bathes

the bodies of the deceased, dresses
each one in clothing brought
by loved ones, sets their hands

and combs their hair, placing them
in caskets their families will never open,
and the mounting waves of sorrow

swell high and higher, until they crest
and the rushing waters wash,
and wash, and wash over him.

## HOBOKEN, NOVEMBER 2020

We missed the eruption,
the cheers and applause,

the revved engines and car horns,
but the late afternoon air

was still abuzz when my daughters
and I walked ten electric blocks

down Washington Street, weaving
through clusters of glowing celebrants,

and around tables full of diners
lingering over a drink or bite

in the unseasonal warmth of that November
day. One daughter suggested we find

another route to skirt the crowds,
to spare my energy as we wended our way

to the bookstore. I shrugged off the idea,
fatigued in body but energized

by the reverberation of hope on that
crowded city street after months

and years of our nation's silent despair.
A young mother holding the hand

of her small child, a girl, three or four
years old, slowed to tilt her head downward

as my daughters and I walked past.
The mother leaned in to her daughter

and said, *Kamala. Her name is Kamala.*

## IN STATE

America is lying in state today,
laid bare in this consecrated place
where she fought against her ravaging

four years ago, where she cried
and shook through her death throes,
as we turned away, away,

and, again, away. Here, the fury
of a jilted man caught the wind,
as it always does, and poisoned

our nation's imagination,
until we could no longer see
what we know we all saw.

America is lying in state today,
in this sacred place of the people
where past commanders rested,

laid out under the guard
of a flag bowing in gratitude,
under the watch of a nation in grief.

The remains of America are laid
before us, here in the Rotunda,
at the feet of a flaccid man beholden

to the spectacle of pomp without circumstance,
of a lowered flag ordered to stand
without consent and without respect, at full mast.

Together, we mourn our beloved stars
and stripes, limp and shuddering, sad
witness to our nation's blustering death rattle.

# THE ALCHEMY OF CRISIS

Rage broils just below my skin,
layered between despair and turmoil.

I want to slip a butterfly needle
under the thin dermal sheath,

pull back the plunger and drain
the hot fluid built up and ready

to bubble over. Instead, words seep
from my fingers onto the page,

loosen the grief until it softens and flows,
banking on alchemy that they arrive

in your ear as resistance,
as hope. We will not back down.

# HEALTH CARE PROXY

I am grateful for the red light
a few blocks from St. Luke's,

the minute or two it offers, for lifting
my phone from the dashboard mount,

for opening the email, heart pounding,
hands shaking. I need to be ready.

At the empty intersection on a clear November day,
I find the attorney's message, download

the attachment, scroll to paragraph II, section B,
as directed by my brother across the country.

There it is, laid out in clear language –
there were to be no lifesaving measures.

No CPR, no assisted breathing, no
nothing.

I did not know.
Nobody knew.

When the light turns, I lift my foot
move forward on the quiet street, breathe

fast, deep, my chest heaving. The end is clear.
The hospital sign ahead glares bright in the midday sun.

I circle the full parking lot, fast, searching.
I give up, pull into a spot on the street, unsure

if it is legal, not pausing to check.
Caught in a tangle of seatbelt and bags,

I try to free myself from the car, grab
my laptop, notepad, water bottle.

Everything falls to the floor.
I stuff it all, whatever I can scoop up

in one sweep, back into my tote.
I slam the car door, run-walk to the entrance,

push through the revolving door, make a beeline
down the hall to a bathroom,

pull the door closed, fumble with my zipper.
I barely make it before my bladder voids.

So this is how shock, grief, and despair,
all work together, unleashed within the body.

What else will sorrow shake loose, on the other
side of the hospital room door?

I give myself a minute to cry,
knowing what is to come,

now that we no longer hold the luxury
of time or faith in miracles.

A shudder rocks through me,
shoulders to tailbone.

I straighten my spine, approach
the security desk, and ask for the room

in the ICU where my brother lies unconscious,
on a ventilator, alive but dying.

In the elevator to the 4th floor, I brace to tell
my waiting family he does not want any of this.

# TIDAL FORCES

Hurricane Gloria lashed and churned
over my New England hometown

on my father's birthday when I was fifteen,
and I walked onto the stone jetty at the beach

with my brother. I can feel the push
and pull of gale forces against my thin

body still, water spraying from ocean
and sky at once, my flapping clothes damp

and heavy, coated in a mist of wet sand.
I trusted my brother. But we should not

have been standing on that rocky pier,
as waves crashed at our feet and the hurricane

roiled around us, flooded streets and splintered
boats. Now, I question his judgment, imagine

how fast we might be swept into the swell.
My mother would have been distressed

had she known he took me into the heart
of the storm. But we made it home that day,

with blurry photos to mark our victory.
It was another forty years before a storm

barreled through my brother's body,
sent him tumbling to his death.

I stand here in the wake, reeling
from the force of it all.

## TAX SEASON

I find you there, in the tally
of my year –

in spring –
my new book you paid for through Paypal,
a family vacation with all of us siblings
and our inexplicable fallout

in summer –
your silence, the calls
I did not make

in fall –
all the miles to Massachusetts logged,
so nearby but not there
for your birthday,
and again, the week before
your fall

at year's end –
you appear once more
in my ledger –
gas and tolls, 95 North to 195,
highway coffee stops,

then a projector, easels, audio supplies
ordered online, photos printed at CVS,
your funeral cards designed
and paid for in Jersey –

each quiet line item –
a mark of your absence.

# SPRING MORNING

The fetal lambs were alive
but dying, their birth struggle
too strong for the mother.

Her heavy, heaving body
wore out after hours of labor,
went slack, but did not go still.

He vowed to never raise sheep again.

Her swollen belly kept rippling
through the night as her babies
kicked and clamored, but could not

find their way out. My brother wept
as he massaged the ewe's belly,
but by morning they were gone.

All of them.

# ASSISTED BREATHING

*Put on your own oxygen mask*
*first.*

For years, I dispensed this snappy
wisdom to myself and to friends lost

in the sleepless nights, the conflicted
allegiances of parenting.

This was before people spoke of self-care.
Back then, we were in survival mode.

Back then, we needed to remind ourselves
to breathe. But it wasn't literal.

Nobody actually had an oxygen mask.
Life has grown more fragile.

When the air became thin,
my mask went on first.

The message – *stay alive so you can help*
*your children* – still holds true.

It's no longer a metaphor.
And I did    and I am.

## AFTER THE BOOK FAIR, NEW JERSEY CITY UNIVERSITY

A day like today is filled with wonder,
of students offering books to other students,

of poets putting words into the air, of people
making plans for tomorrow. The wonder

is not there alone. The awe that fuels
my body today is that love is given here, now,

amid despair and chaos, amid crisis. So I know,
our imaginations will not be stripped

bare in tandem with our freedoms.
We will make our way through, together.

# PAPER TRAILS

Pages float through the night sky
on the New Jersey Turnpike,

fluttering in the glow of headlights
reflecting off the glistening roadbed.

Words aloft, drift on the air.
The unknown composer travels

away, away, leaving a trail
of missives in their silent wake.

Tomorrow, people will open
front doors to damp sheets

of paper plastered on steps,
caught in high branches, peeking

from flower beds. Who will pause
to claim these lines launched

into the wind—stray remains
of an unfinished story?

## HOW TO END

A fellow writer once advised,
come evening, always stop
on the downhill.
End the day's work gliding
through paragraphs,
slicing sentences right, left, right.
Fast and smooth.

And then, stop.
Just stop.

Offer the gift of an easy start
to the writer
you will be tomorrow.

# FAILURE

I slept last night to the drumbeat
of heavy rain, woke to the sound

of tires pulling water from asphalt
as cars passed down the street outside

my window, saw photos on my phone
of mid-April snowfall to the west

and to the north, thought why not,
turned over and closed my eyes again.

A few hours later, the rain slowed
to a cold drip, the cat who waits

for me each morning was sitting
on the table outside my backdoor,

looking in the window at me,
hungry for her breakfast.

## HOW I LIVE NOW

If I extend my gaze outward
from the pain held within

this small body, I may collapse
from the enormity of our grief.

# BENDING TOWARD HOPE

A woman I've never met before –
a stranger, but also, soon,

a confidante – starts by telling
me she has good luck.

Before sharing her story, of cancer
and its recurrence, she needs

to establish this baseline truth
to remind herself,

and so I know to listen
with an ear bent toward hope.

# ACKNOWLEDGEMENTS

*Autumn Sky Poetry Daily:* "Kindred"
*By the WAYE:* "Upon Reflection on the Spring Calendar"
*Eunoia Review:* "Spring Morning"
*Feral:* "Love Note"
*Halfway Down the Stairs:* "Clear Cut"
*MockingHeart Review:* "Reserves"
*New Verse News:* "How to Handle a Leak"
*Nixes Mate Review:* "Tidal Forces"
*One Art:* "Assisted Breathing," "Cleared to Leave," "Emergency Room Visits in March 2020," "In Anticipation of an Elegy," "The Funeral Director, Spring 2020," and "Bending Toward Hope"
*Pangyrus LitMag:* "The Day Another Gun Law Is Repealed"
*Paterson Literary Review:* "A Final Offering"
*Red Eft Review:* "When the Forsythia Blooms"
*The Nature of Our Times:* "September Walk in the New Jersey Pine Barrens after Hurricane Helene"
*Thimble Literary Magazine:* "Tendrils"
*Second Coming:* "After the Book Fair, New Jersey City University" and "The Alchemy of Crisis"
*Silver Birch Press:* "The Baker" and "Lesson in Care" (originally published as "Raccoons in the Attic")
*Snapdragon: A Journal of Art and Healing:* "How to End"
*Stirring:* "A Small Respite" (originally published as "Of Grace and Silence")
*Wild Roof Journal:* "The sky in my backyard is opening"

I owe my deepest gratitude to the communities and people who have sustained and supported me as a poet. Here are but a few of them.

To Anne Elezabeth Pluto and Michael McInnis at Nixes Mate Books for accepting this book and shepherding it with care and patience into the world.

To Jennifer Franklin and the rotating members of our Tuesday night poetry class under whose generosity and care this book took shape –Anne Elezabeth Pluto, Lynne Shapiro, Jonathan Blunk, Tzynya Pinchback, Christy Prahl, Roseann English, Ann Hostetler, Katherine Dering, Lisa Schapiro, Carol Dorf, Elizabeth Falcon, Gail Donahue.

To my WildStory podcast partner, Kim Correro and to all of our guests who have inspired me with their wisdom, their work, and their words.

To my steadfast Sunday morning Colgate crew – Jennifer R. Edwards, Christina Kelly, Michael Foran, Thomas Frank, David Harris.

To James Crews, Sean Thomas Dougherty and Rebecca Hart Olander for supporting this collection with thoughtfulness and care.

And, as always, to Konstantin, Molly, Connie, and Katia, and to my parents Janet and Vern Wallace.

I offer this book in memory of my brother Christopher John Wallace.

## ABOUT THE AUTHOR

Ann E. Wallace, PhD is Poet Laureate Emeritus of Jersey City, New Jersey. As a long-time survivor of ovarian cancer, a woman with multiple sclerosis, and one of the nation's first Long Covid patients, she has lived and written through illness for more than thirty years. Pain, disability, and disease – as well as hope and resilience – have inspired and informed her work as a poet, memoirist, patient advocate, and scholar. Wallace's previous poetry collections include *Days of Grace and Silence: A Chronicle of COVID's Long Haul* (Kelsay Books) and *Counting by Sevens* (Main Street Rag). Her work is included in *The Nature of Our Times* (Paloma Press), *The Big Brutal Act Anthology* (Harbor Anthologies), and *Literacy and Learning in Times of Crisis: Emergent Teaching through Emergencies* (Peter Lang), and her essays have appeared in *Huffington Post*, *USA Today*, *WSQ*, and elsewhere.

An avid gardener, Wallace is co-host and co-producer of *The WildStory: A Podcast of Poetry and Plants* by the Native Plant Society of New Jersey. She grew up in Marion, Massachusetts, and migrated many years ago to New Jersey to study art at Drew University. She holds a master's degree in Women's Studies from Rutgers University and a doctorate in English Literature from The Graduate Center of The City University of New York and is Professor of English at New Jersey City University. Find her online at AnnWallacePhD.com.

# 42° 19' 47.9" N · 70° 56' 43.9" W

Nixes Mate is a navigational hazard in Boston Harbor used during the colonial period to gibbet and hang pirates and mutineers.

Nixes Mate Books features small-batch artisanal literature, created by writers who use all 26 letters of the alphabet and then some, honing their craft the time-honored way: one line at a time.

nixesmate.pub

www.ingramcontent.com/pod-product-compliance
Lightning Source LLC
Chambersburg PA
CBHW060536080526
44586CB00012B/754